When Food Is Your Drug

A Food Addict's Guide to

Managing Emotional Eating

Kristin Jones

ISBN: 978-1-09147-135-1

Dedication

To my parents, Cathy and Richard Jones, for having the patience, faith and trust in me even when I didn't have it in myself. As much as I caused you hours of worry, you never gave up on me and were there with love and support throughout all my challenges.

Grandma, you are my best friend and the one constant in my life when all other things are chaotic. Thank you for loving me with all your heart, no matter what.

You are unconditional love.

Poppy, you are far and away the most loyal, honorable and committed person I will ever know in my life and all of my best qualities, I got from you. Thank you for letting me be such a big part of your life these past few years. We have come a long way, and I love you so much.

Contents

Introduction

I wish I had been a drug addict.

No, seriously. Life would be so much easier as a meth or crack head. You get hooked on one of those substances and you just know your life is heading for the shitter, and it becomes pretty obvious to those around you that you have a problem as well.

You lose your job. Stop caring for your personal hygiene. Beg, borrow and steal from those you love in order to get your next fix.

When you finally hit rock bottom, the intervention is done and you are loaded into a van and whisked away to a facility in southern Florida, you know that after your stint in rehab you will return to your life and have to make some big changes... the biggest being completely eliminating the negative influences—people, circumstances and surroundings—from your life in order for you to make a clean break and start your life moving in a new and positive direction.

But when food is your drug of choice, that is just not possible.

Drugs and alcohol are not substances we need to survive. They are known toxins that create havoc and chaos in the lives of people who choose to partake in them. Food doesn't work that way. You don't have a choice... you *have to eat*. You can't eliminate it from your life any more than you can eliminate water and expect to last longer than three days.

Food issues are far and away the hardest form of addiction to give up and recover from. In reality, just like someone who abuses drugs or alcohol, a food issue never goes away. You are always in recovery, trying to learn to deal with the feelings and emotions that drive you to behaviors that don't serve you. It does not become about eliminating the problem but learning to manage it. When I learned this fact from my therapist, Mary Gail, I was simultaneously pissed and relieved.

I thought, "Oh, crap. This is *never* going away?"

But then suddenly, I felt an overwhelming sense of relief when I realized that it wasn't that I just sucked and couldn't get over this myself. No matter what I did, these feelings were always going to be there, and it became all about how I responded and dealt with them that made the difference.

You probably didn't pick up this book thinking you were going to be compared to a drug user, but the reality is this: If you are either unable to lose weight, even with the best of intentions, or you have lost and gained the same 20 pounds at least ten times and you just can't figure out why it keeps coming back, you are doing the same dance with food that an addict does with drugs. Or an alcoholic does with vodka.

Nine-year-old girls, when asked what they want to be when they grow up, don't say, "I want to be a druggie." No one wants that for themselves or anyone they love. Just the same as you didn't say at nine years old, "When I grow up, I want to have issues with food that will keep me overweight, unhappy and feeling ashamed and disappointed with myself for the rest of my life."

I didn't want that, and I am quite sure you didn't want that either, but that's where we ended up through no fault of our own. But here you are, grown up and adulting, and it is time to make a choice.

Do you keep doing what you are doing and hope that somehow the next diet works and you lose the weight, keep it off and your life magically falls perfectly into place?

Or do you decide to take a look at the persistent underlying issues that surround why you can't lose weight and keep it off, do the work to learn how to respond to these issues, and then move on with your life and let food have its appropriate place in your life?

(That means not being the center of your life.)

If that is why you picked up this book, you are in the right place. You will be asked to do something that is surprisingly simple yet incredibly hard. You are going to have to look at your emotions and how you express them—or don't express them—and how that simple act has altered the trajectory of your life and left you with 10, 20 or even 100 pounds to lose and a hole in your heart from the pain, anguish and disappointment you have felt after each time you have tried to lose the weight yourself and failed miserably.

I have spent most of my life completely obsessed with food, my appearance and what others think of me based upon what I look like. It started so early for me that I never even thought I could go through a day, or even an hour of my day, without thoughts that focused on what I was going to eat next and what the impact would be on my body. The anxiety, discomfort, shame and disappointment I felt on an hourly basis proved exhausting and overwhelming... but those emotions served a purpose. They protected me from having to address and deal with emotions and beliefs that I just didn't feel I was strong enough to deal with. I have learned that I am strong enough, smart enough and empowered enough to face, head on, these thoughts, and that I have the power within me to know who I am based upon me and not what others have told me I am.

My hope is for you to know that you can do this, too, and that through reading this book and doing the work that goes along with it, you will be able to recognize, embrace and love who you really are and know you are perfect just the way you are regardless of your upbringing, or labels, or beliefs others have put upon you.

Approach reading this book in the same way a doctor would go about treating a medical condition like a skin rash. Acknowledge the current situation, look at the symptoms and know they are merely what is on the surface and that there is something deeper going on. Think back to when you believe the symptoms originated, determine what caused them and figure out what behavior changes need to occur in order for the situation to not present itself again. Then, formulate a plan so you can avoid this condition in the future.

Have a journal or notebook dedicated to the writing activities outlined in this book and really take your time when completing these "assignments." I was a middle school teacher for 17 years and spent nine of them working with children with learning disabilities, and I know all about brain research and the process of retaining information. The act of thinking a thought and then the process it takes to put it to paper helps to imprint the information on the brain and then allows it to be recalled and readily used.

Sometimes it's easier to take a very clinical approach to addressing deep-seated emotional issues and if that works for you, please go about it this way. Know how brave, courageous, strong and tenacious you are for confronting your unhealthy relationship with food, and know that things can and will be different for you by following the steps outlined in this book.

One caveat that I feel I must mention...If, while you read this book and begin to uncover deeply personal and emotional circumstances in your life, you feel overwhelmed by your thoughts and feelings, please know that professional help is just a phone call away. There are so many amazingly kind, understanding and knowledgeable therapists who can help you work through what you have uncovered and can help you address and work on moving past unhealed emotional trauma. Please seek professional help for more direct and personal care.

I am excited for you as you embark on this journey of self-discovery and know that freedom from emotional eating is possible.

Will it happen automatically just because you read this book?

No.

Will it require vulnerability and honesty, the likes of which you might never have allowed yourself to experience in your entire life?

Absolutely.

Please believe me when I say that the work, discomfort, effort and vulnerability is all worth it for the peace, serenity and joy that awaits you once you have dealt with your emotional eating. It is so incredible, and I want that for you more than I can express.

Be patient with yourself and know that it won't happen overnight. With persistent focus and dedication, you will have a healthy relationship with food, and it will carry over to all aspects of your life.

Chapter 1
Putting a Name to It

Mayonnaise is my kryptonite. Put it on french fries, pizza, a peanut butter sandwich... there is nothing that is not improved with a bit of mayo. Once I start indulging, the wheels come off and I have no control over the food choices I make from that point on.

Hungry or not.

Full and bordering on uncomfortable, I will continue eating if mayonnaise is part of the equation. I become weak and unable to use my better judgement to steer away from eating it on anything.

Hi, my name is Kristin, and I am an emotional eater.

Although a constant challenge to deal with, my unhealthy focus on image and weight has proven to be a blessing because it has fueled my desire to help others, like you, in dealing with body image issues.

Just like me, I know you desperately want to be healthy and happy with your body but find life overwhelming. Things feel out of control, especially where food is concerned, and you think if you could just get that under control, all would fall into place.

I know a great deal about wanting to—and needing to—keep control of all aspects of life. When you suffer from an eating disorder, it's not about the foods you are eating, or not eating, but the perception of control you want over your thoughts, emotions and surroundings... every aspect of your life. All you want is for life to be settled, calm, and for you to have a feeling of control.

So you try every kind of diet that comes along to see if "this one" is going to be the magic bullet that will not only melt the fat away, but wash away the disappointment and disgust you feel on a daily basis. You have lost control because your body isn't the way you want it to be, and you aren't helping the situation because of what you are doing.

If you feel like you are all alone in these feelings, rest assured that you are NOT the only one. And by picking up this book, you are brave enough to want to do something about it.

Does Any of This Sound Familiar?

Do you get up in the morning, stand on your scale and swear it must be stuck? Or that the gravitational pull in your bathroom is stronger than the rest of the planet?

Do you stand in front of the mirror, grab your muffin top and swear and curse under your breath that you've JUST GOT TO lose weight?

Do you struggle to pull up your pants and secure the button, all the while praying to the pant gods that it holds until you get home from work?

Do you analyze and criticize every morsel of food that passes your lips?

Do you berate yourself for not having the self-control and self-discipline to make the right decisions about what you eat?

Do you feel you have no control around food, or situations involving food?

You want to stick with a routine and see results, but it just isn't happening. Career, kids and life responsibilities take over and your needs are at the bottom of the list.

Suddenly, you're exhausted, disappointed and frustrated, and you don't know where to turn.

I know that pain. It has been my companion and friend. I have lived it in one iteration or another for most of my life.

Waking up with that nauseated feeling because I just couldn't go to bed without eating that last bite of ice cream or just one more cookie... for some reason feeling like if I didn't eat it then, in that very moment, I was not going to make it through the night. That feeling of anxiety and nervousness I believed could only be remedied with just one more bite of food.

This book has been written to help you realize if emotional eating is a problem for you, and it will also provide you with proven steps and strategies to help you learn to embrace this part of yourself, love it unconditionally and learn how to manage difficult situations instead of turning to food.

For years and years, I believed I was the only one who ever had these feelings, and I rationalized them as just what I did (so, normal for me although in my heart I knew something was "off"), but they weren't something I could share or let anyone else witness. Others would surely think I was crazy, weird or even worse, unlovable. So, I worked very hard to keep these traits a secret from family, friends and co-workers, and spent an exorbitant amount of time obsessing over how I interacted with food.

Characteristics of an Emotional Eater

What does it mean to be an emotional eater? I started my unhealthy relationship with food when I was probably five years old, but it didn't kick into full-blown eating disorder mode until I started dieting obsessively at the age of 16. Then it took me another 18 years to actually be able to own the label of having an eating disorder.

I remember it like it was yesterday...

Sixteen years old and sitting on the kitchen counter in a room filled with relatives. I jumped off the counter and when I landed with a thud, my uncle made a comment for everyone in the room to hear:

"Better be careful or you might break the floor next time you jump off the counter like that."

I pretended to laugh it off, but this was the beginning of a downward spiral.

That one innocent comment struck a deep chord within me, but the thing is, this is not when my issues with food and my weight started... that seed had been planted years before and it was slowly growing, infiltrating every aspect of my being and eating away at my self-worth and esteem. This incident just started the "launch sequence" that could not be aborted, and the result was an eating disorder that would turn into a lifelong battle.

Why did it take me so long to acknowledge that I had an eating disorder? There is so much shame and embarrassment that goes along with having any kind of addiction, and to think that you can't control yourself around food is just humiliating. What? Are you kidding me? It is a part of everyday life... something you have to do to survive, and you can't pull your head out of your ass long enough to be able to know when you should eat and when you shouldn't?

In my mind, you had to be all kinds of fucked up to not be able to manage that.

I didn't fall into the well-known categories of eating disorders, anorexia and bulimia, but I always knew there was something very unhealthy and destructive about my relationship with food and couldn't name it. It wasn't until very recently that the term "emotional eating" kept coming on my radar, and the term resonated with me immediately.

As I go through the typical characteristics of an emotional eater, pay attention to whether I am painting a picture of what might describe you and your behaviors. I can only speak for myself, but I found it incredibly freeing and liberating to be able to give a name to these behaviors I had sought to hide from the world, and myself, for so many years. It gave me a sense of peace to know that I was not the only one who felt this way or did these things.

An emotional eater is a person who finds them selves eating when they are not experiencing physical hunger, one who oftentimes has a difficult time stopping themselves from eating even if they are full. Whether alone or in social situations, they feel powerless over food and find it almost impossible to not give into their cravings. Cravings for certain types of foods lead many down the road of emotional eating, and ignoring cravings is just not an option.

Emotional eaters find it next to impossible to differentiate between physical and emotional hunger. This is a huge issue that prevents many individuals from being able to even recognize they have an issue with food. They complain of always being hungry, but the reality is that they really are not.

Emotional Hunger vs. Physical Hunger

Physical hunger and emotional hunger may appear very similar, but there are key differences between the two and it is important to focus on what you are feeling in order to distinguish between the two sensations.

Physical hunger grows slowly and is satisfied by any kind of food, whereas emotional hunger comes on suddenly and only sugary junk foods that provide an instant rush to the system, will do. Mindlessly eating is a sign of emotional hunger, and individuals with emotional eating issues will often not even remember what they have eaten due to "checking out" while eating (Smith, Segal, & Segal, 2018; link: https://www.

helpguide.org/articles/diets/emotional-
eating.htm).

Emotional hunger is not satisfied even when a person is full; their head is dictating whether they are satisfied and usually that results in eating past the point of satisfaction. When this point is reached, an emotional eater will experience feelings of extreme shame, guilt and disappointment in themselves and their behaviors. When a person is meeting physical hunger, they are able to eat what they need, stop when satisfied and not feel any sensations of guilt (Smith et al, 2018; link: https://www. helpguide.org/articles/diets/emotional-eating.htm).

Does any of this sound familiar?

The first step in tackling a difficult life situation is acknowledging there is a problem and processing what that means to you and how it makes you feel. Throughout this book, I am going to ask you to think about certain scenarios and questions that will allow you to dive in to your emotions and what you are truly feeling about your life and circumstances. In order to make any progress in learning to deal with emotional eating, you must be willing to strip away your protective armor and look at the choices you've made in the past. I am not asking you to tear yourself apart emotionally, but I *do* ask that you be honest about what defense mechanisms you have used in the past to get you through situations.

Please have a composition or spiral notebook with you while reading this book, because I will ask you to write about certain scenarios and circumstances from your own life. My hope is that this might help you develop an understanding of your own unique situation. I find that when I put things in writing, they become much more real and tangible for me, and I am better able to make sense of them.

Answer the following questions as honestly as you can. The first step in overcoming any situation or circumstance is total transparency and honesty. For each question you answer with a "yes", please write that question as a statement in your notebook. Example: "I absolutely eat when I am not hungry, or when I am full." Be real with yourself. Now is the time.

Are You an Emotional Eater?

- **Do you eat more when stressed?**

- **Do you eat when you are not hungry, or when you're full?**

- **Do you eat to feel better (when you're mad, bored, anxious, etc.)?**

- **Do you reward yourself with food?**

- **Do you regularly eat until you are stuffed?**

- **Does food make you feel safe?**

- **Do you feel like food is your friend?**

- **Do you feel powerless or out of control around food?**

(Smith et al, 2018; link: https://www.helpguide.org/articles/diets/emotional-eating.htm)

Even answering just one of these questions with a "yes" could indicate that food has an unbalanced, or unhealthy, impact on your life that might not be serving you in a positive way.

Stop and Jot #1

For any of the questions you answered "yes" to and wrote as a declarative statement in your journal, please write about the situation and how you used this coping mechanism. Write as much as you can for each statement. Don't edit yourself, just put your thoughts to paper and get them out of your head.

Behaviors of an Emotional Eater

What does it look like to be an emotional eater? Do you have to be 10, 20, 50 pounds overweight? Do you walk around with food scraps attached to the front of your sweater indicating an emotional eating session has just concluded?

No, emotional eaters are masters at disguising their behaviors, but more specifically their feelings, so there is not a stereotype of what an emotional eater looks like. Many share similar behaviors that are challenging to manage, but they will do anything to "manage" them as best they can so that no one is able to figure out what is truly going on.

I am a perfect example. If anyone were to look at me, they would never in a million years think I have issues with food. I am tall and thin, with well-defined arms and a narrow waist... not what you would expect from a person who can polish off a half a loaf of French bread slathered in mayonnaise without blinking an eye. Yes, I said mayonnaise, and it is my weakness. I should weigh three times what I weigh, but to go along with my emotional eating, I have learned coping skills to overcome and balance out the damage I do to my body through my eating.

Emotional eating may be an issue for you if you:

- **Eat in secret.** I must have gone close to six months without letting anyone see me eat anything. I can't tell you how often people would say, "Kristin never eats anything." Ha!

- **Are defensive about what you eat and how much.** During the rare times I *did* eat in front of others, I was often interrogated over what I was eating. I hate being the center of attention, and when the spotlight fell on me and what I was eating, it reaffirmed to me why I should never eat in front of others.

- **Avoid social situations due to fear of not being able to control the foods present.** Isn't it normal to go online and preview the menu at a restaurant to ensure that there is something "safe" you can eat in front of others? Or bring your own food to restaurants since you know what is in the meal you have prepared? Doesn't everybody do that? What? No? Oh, I guess it was just me.

- **Constantly think about food and what you are going to eat next.** There is so much information on the Internet that it's easy to obsess over every morsel of food you put into your mouth. How many calories? Fat grams? Too many carbs? Not enough protein? It becomes a full-time job for some emotional eaters, and one with a huge price to pay.

- **Elimination of certain food groups.** This is a common strategy used by emotional eaters to help them regain some sense of control over their crazy world of food. I have done this too many times to count. One week I was vegan, then the next I was high carb/low-fat, then gluten-free...all a thinly veiled attempt to justify making foods forbidden in an attempt to keep them under control.

- **Anger/jealousy toward "normal" eaters.** Nothing would make me more upset than to see a thin person saddle up to a table full of delicious treats, take a little bit of each thing, taste everything and then throw away what they didn't finish. WTF? Throw away food? Blasphemy! Not in my world. I wanted to know their secret... and now I do and will share it with you soon enough.

Does any of the above resonate with you? Do you see any of these behaviors in yourself? Are you exhausted trying to keep all your "food balls" in the air, trying to preserve the impression that you have your world under control?

Okay, so what? I am an emotional eater, is that really so bad? What is the collateral damage of this unhealthy relationship?

Aftermath of Emotional Eating

The first and most obvious result of emotional eating is the inability to either lose or maintain any kind of weight loss. Consistent episodes of eating beyond feelings of fullness will definitely impact a person's overall calorie consumption and result in weight gain. If you are actively trying to lose weight and you consistently sabotage your efforts by eating when it is not necessary, the shame and disgust you feel toward yourself is way more damaging than the foods you eat and the effect they have on your body. Yes, weight gain can have troubling consequences if left unattended, but the damage each of us inflicts upon ourselves through negative self-talk is even more destructive and can leave wounds that never heal, exacerbating the cycle of disappointment and guilt which often results in more emotional eating.

When things in your life are not going how you would like them to, it is easy to want to hide from others and avoid dealing with your issues, whatever they may be. In the case of emotional eating, the absence of control causes many eaters to isolate themselves from others because it is too painful to have to deal with the awkward social situations that often accompany food. This alienation can make a person even more sad and hopeless, and in turn can cause emotional eating to occur. Again, another vicious cycle.

Emotional eaters view food as an escape; a place of refuge in an ever-chaotic world that allows focusing on something other than a problem or issue. Instead of dealing with why you were fired from your job, why not just buy a pizza and eat it all in one sitting? Don't want to deal with your loveless marriage? A pint of Ben and Jerry's can definitely take the edge off that yearning you've had for months. Food becomes a distraction, or in many cases, an obsession, that allows a person to disengage from their feelings and find temporary comfort.

And lastly, the shame, disappointment and disgust felt after eating way beyond the point of satisfaction cannot be fully understood unless you have been there and know what that feels like. This feeling of letting yourself down, and the disparaging comments you make to yourself hurt your heart more than words or actions anyone else could ever say or do to you. Not only do you have these feelings toward yourself, you compound the problem by verbally assaulting your character and the very essence of your being with hurtful messages that tear you down at your very core. Far and away, the most destructive and abusive person in your life is often the one you see in the mirror.

Numerous studies have shown how negative self-talk can impact overall health and outlook on life. Higher stress levels, lower self-esteem and a lack of internal motivation are likely present in someone who engages in belittling themselves and sabotaging their own progress by speaking poorly of themselves (Scalise, 2018; link: https://brainspeak.com/how-negative-self-talk-sabotages-your-health-happiness/). More stress results in an increase in the production of cortisol, the belly fat hormone, and this can impact weight-loss efforts and cause more negative self-talk.

Where to Now?

Okay, so you now know what it means to have an emotional issue with food, how it can present itself and the results that alter your life in so many ways. You also should be able to confidently say whether the label of "Emotional Eater" applies to you. Again, I want to emphasize the relief I felt once I was able to give the patterns I had developed over my lifetime of food issues a name and recognized that I was not the only one who did these types of things.

By being able to acknowledge the behaviors, I was then able to address them in a way that did not threaten my self-confidence...in fact, knowing my problem led me to be able to take the steps needed to deal with it.

You might notice I never use phrases like, "learn to overcome your issues with food" or "ways to fix your emotional eating patterns," and that is very deliberate. The most important thing I learned in my third round of therapy (finally found a therapist I really connected with) regarding my issues with food was the idea that it is just like being an alcoholic. It is not something that will ever "go away" or that you will "fix", it is part of who you are, and you will never be without these feelings.

I had come into a session with my therapist, and I was again sharing with her another episode of out-of-control eating. I remember so clearly, like it was yesterday, pleading with her, "What is wrong with me? When is this going to go away? Why can't I just GET IT?"

And in a calm, controlled way, she clearly stated the words that changed my life, and this was the first step in healing my issues with food.

She said, "Kristin, this is never going to go away. It is part of who you are at your very core, and the sooner you learn to love this part of yourself, the easier things will get. It is not about 'fixing the issue,' but it *is* about learning how to respond to the emotions that come up in a way that lessens the impact it has on your self-esteem and your viewpoint of yourself."

What? It is *never going away*?

I was pissed at first, but only for a brief moment, because then I realized that there wasn't anything wrong with me. Instead, I just had strategies to learn that would allow me to live life "normally" and have a healthy relationship with food.

I am the type of person who loves to be able to solve my own problems, so this became my rallying cry: I am not going to "fix" myself, but I am going to do everything I can do to make sure I know how to react to my feelings toward food.

Now, because of this breakthrough did I suddenly know exactly what to do and how to talk to myself when I started getting weird with food? Oh heck no, it was many years later that I truly learned where all my issues with food came from and what I really needed to do to address them. And that is what we are going to talk about next.

Author's Note:

Please keep in mind that the issues you are dealing with in your life might not present themselves in the same way mine do, and of course, that is what makes each of us unique. In fact, you might not have an issue with food, but instead it might be an issue with wine, exercise, prescription drugs, online gaming or recreational drugs. Whatever it is that you use to detach and remove yourself from the challenging emotions you have in your life, everything I talk about in this book can be applied to those substances or processes. Keep reading and you will be able to take your "vice" and go through the same steps in order to learn the strategies and process needed to embrace this part of who you are.

Chapter 2
How Did I Get Here?

I was blessed to grow up having close relationships with both sets of grandparents: My dad's parents, Nona and Papa, and my mom's mom, Grandma. Through these connections, I was able to learn how important family was and how you value your family over all else.

As a young child, I loved my family more than anything, but I had no clue about the mass dysfunction that was taking place on both sides of my family due to addiction issues.

Were any of my relatives bad people? Heavens, no.

Did they know how to cope with their feelings and express themselves in healthy and balanced ways? Oh, heck no.

But were they doing the best they could, given the information and the upbringing they had experienced? Of course.

When confronting an issue like emotional eating, it is important to understand where the habits and thought processes you have used to survive originated from. It is also vital to not dwell on what you discover. Investigate, acknowledge, change your perspective and move on with these new tools in place to respond appropriately to any circumstance.

Are you always going to do it correctly? No, but you will have the strategies and information to make an informed decision about how to move forward.

Throughout the remainder of this book, you are going to be asked to "stop and jot" your thoughts, feelings and emotions about certain aspects of your childhood. It is very important that you feel safe doing this and know how vital it is to the process of managing emotional eating. It will be difficult and painful at times, but you must go back through what you dealt with to embrace it, accept it and then change your viewpoint of it, if you ever expect to move past it.

**Always remember that if feelings and emotions start to come up that you feel you don't have control over, and you start to feel overwhelmed, good counseling services are always a fabulous options to help you work through these issues. This book is not a replacement for therapy if you believe that is what you need. My hope is that this book will get you thinking and moving in the right direction to work through and accept the situation you are in and love yourself no matter what.

Stop and Jot #2

Label this journal entry "Emotional Eating Encounters". You are going to write down all the circumstances during which emotional eating takes place.

Things to think about before you begin:

- *Do certain social situations make emotional eating more prevalent?*

- *Does it happen around specific people?*

- *Do family events or interactions cause you anxiety, resulting in overeating?*

- *Does it happen at home?*

- *What action or event precedes an episode, regardless of where it happens?*

- *Can you recall the emotions you felt prior to starting to eat?*

- *Must you be alone?*

Set your timer for two minutes and try to come up with as many situations as you can during which emotional eating occurs. Go!

Once you have this first list, set another minute on the timer and look for common threads or similarities on the list, and group them together, such as "Work Performance", "Disagreements", or "Lonely". This list will be used in a later activity, so please be as exhaustive as you can and go into as much detail as possible.

Back in the late 90s, there were a number of talk shows like Jerry Springer, Geraldo, Sally Jessy Raphael and Maury Povich, and these programs showcased regular people with issues in their lives they wanted to get help with on national television. Not something I would recommend, but to each his own.

These people often had some kind of traumatic early life experience, and the shows would allow these individuals to share their stories and hopefully come to some place of peace about whatever happened in their lives.

More often than not, the entire show was spent with these people looking to place blame on someone in their childhood for messing up their lives instead of taking responsibility for their role in the dysfunction and realizing they could change their perspective regarding everything that happened to them.

Yes, in this book you are going to need to look at things that were said to you, done to you and that you did to others, but what I implore you to do is this one thing: Always remember that everyone—your parents, grandparents and assorted relatives—was doing the best they could with the modeling they received as young children, and no one wants to cause another pain... they just want to alleviate their own pain through whatever means they can.

This is NOT about blaming anyone, especially your parents or caregivers, but instead merely acknowledging where behaviors originated and how they manifested in your life, and then choosing to write a new story about the situation that better serves you in adulthood.

Dad's Food

Nona was an incredible cook and coming from Oklahoma, she made some of the best food I have ever eaten in my life. In a southern home, preparing food is a display of love. That is the environment my dad grew up in, and he knew no other way. Although my mom did not know how to cook early on, Nona taught her the skills she learned at the age of 15 so she could be prepared to be a wife and mother who knew how to show her love for her family through food. Food was a focus and a unifying element in my house growing up, but it also served to divide us and caused me to believe things about myself that were not true.

The beginning of my issues with food started when I was about five years old and I realized there were rules associated with food in our house. My dad had food that was strictly for him and we (my mom, two brothers and my sister) were NOT allowed to consume it. Pepsi-Cola in the glass bottles. Dry-roasted peanuts. Vitamin D milk. Although it was never stated, I interpreted this to mean that I was too fat to be able to eat these foods, and the message I received was I needed to do something about my weight.

Stop and Jot #3

Take a moment to respond to these questions:

- *Were their rules attached to your eating at home?*

- *How were meals administered?*

- *Was mealtime seen as an event?*

- *How did you feel about eating meals when you were young? What emotions did you feel at meal time?*

I also heard that I was NOT okay the way I was, and that I might not be lovable unless I was able to do something about my weight.

Forbidden foods in my house also set me up to begin the habit of eating in secret. It started with me sneaking any of the off-limit items I could get away with eating, but it soon led to most foods being eaten in private. Eating food became something that was risky, so I learned to do it without others knowing. It also became my silent way of rebelling and acting out.

There was one environment in my childhood that stands out to me as being a place where it could not have been more obvious that I didn't fit in, and that I needed to "fix myself" so I would be like everyone else. For me, this place was ballet class. Now, ballet class for five-year-olds is not a strict place, but a way for kids to get familiar with moving their bodies and become comfortable with movement. I remember running from one end of the studio to the other and feeling like I was a large dinosaur crushing all things in its path, including my fellow ballerinas. I can remember these feelings like they happened yesterday, and I begged my mom to take me out of ballet class. I couldn't handle the emotions of isolation, inferiority and disappointment I felt when in class, and I knew I needed to change how big I was compared to the other girls. If I did that, maybe I would be allowed to have some of the forbidden foods, or better yet, I actually might feel like I fit in and wasn't such a source of embarrassment to my dad. Again, super important to know that these things were *never* said directly to me but since there was never an explanation about why there were foods I couldn't eat, I was left to my own devices and created my own story.

Go To Your Room

If there is one thing I know with 100% certainty about my childhood, it is that I was not permitted to express my emotions openly. In fact, showing emotions, especially crying, was not encouraged, so I learned early on that if I was going to be a part of the family, I had to accept that I needed to hide how I felt. I sought to make others happy, not worry about myself and what I needed or wanted and hoped that I would be accepted. As a result, I still fight to make myself and my needs a priority in my life.

I was the youngest of four kids, and I always felt like an outsider. I always felt fear when at home, and a strong sense that I didn't fit in with my siblings. It definitely got better as I got older, but early on, life at home was anything but peaceful. The funny thing is, as adults, I am extremely close with my sister, Katy, and my brother, Otis, (my oldest brother, Kevin, died in 2003 from alcoholism) but boy, did we not get along when we all lived together.

Now, as I stated at the beginning of the chapter, this is not about pointing fingers, but rather about finding out where my feelings of insecurity and loneliness came from. In another session of therapy with Mary Gail, we uncovered where my fear of abandonment came from. For as long as I can remember, I always had pretty intense separation anxiety relating to my mom, and I just couldn't figure out why. I knew it was impacting my adult relationships, and I needed to get to the bottom of it.

From the time I was old enough to sleep in a bed, my sister and I shared a bedroom. We lived in a small house in Lafayette, California, and my two brothers shared a room, and Katy and I did as well. When we moved to a larger, two-story house near the Martinez/Pleasant Hill border, my parents were worried about me being upstairs with my sister and their master bedroom being on the first floor. To ease their minds, keep me safe and close to them, they put a small twin bed in a tiny closet right outside of their bedroom, and that is where I slept, alone, scared and without my sister for two years. Little did they know that I felt such incredible abandonment and as a result soon turned to food as a source of comfort since there was no other way to express these feelings of confusion over why my sister had left me all alone.

My mom and I have talked about this, and of course, she and my dad only had my best interests in mind when they made the decision to move me closer to them. They had no idea the effect it would have on me, and this again is another example of parents doing what they think is the right thing and having no ill intent.

Abandonment and isolation are two actions that result in emotions that many people don't want to address or be confronted with. Avoidance, distraction and ignorance are ways to respond, and the use of an addictive substance, or an addictive process, makes doing any of these things so much easier.

The most defining statement made in my child-hood and the one thing I know that has contributed the most to my issues with food and interpersonal relationships was, "If you are going to be like *that,* go to your room or I'll give you something to cry about." The power in this message was devastating to a six-or seven-year-old girl who thought she was fat, that her dad didn't love her and who had constant feelings of separation anxiety as a result of feeling abandoned.

First, it was not okay to display that I was unhappy and make others feel that way as well. Next, if I was going to be weak and show these emotions, I was going to be ostracized from the group and denied the attention or nurturing I really was asking for. I learned very quick that I shouldn't let anyone see how I really felt, and it was not safe to express emotions that might make others uncomfortable. I could be uncomfortable, but I couldn't force how I was feeling onto other people. Everyone's needs were placed ahead of mine.

The second part of this statement is the soul-crushing part of the phrase, and it is a combination of a threat and sucker punch to the gut. The phrase, "or I'll give you something to cry about," was telling me that what I was feeling in that moment, the emotions I had that were not being appropriately hidden, were not legitimate or valid, and that if I didn't stop being so dramatic, something would happen to me that would result in me being legitimately upset. Did I know what that would look like? No, but I also didn't ever push it beyond this point to find out. I took my father's words as credible and sulked back to my room, shut the door and screamed and cried into a pillow, wishing that someday this would all go away.

It was in these lonely moments, when no one came in to check on me and give me the chance to say how I was feeling, right or wrong, that the need for comfort, safety, and love came from, and was the genesis of me turning to food to get the positive feelings I was missing.

Stop and Jot #4

Set your timer for 10 minutes and write as much as you can. Don't censor.

- *How were emotions expressed in your home when you were a child?*

- *Were you, as a child, allowed to freely express yourself?*

- *Do you recall any family member or friend saying something to you about your weight or your eating habits or patterns?*

Conditional Love

I never knew unconditional love. In fact, I never knew it was even a "thing" until I was in my mid-20s when again, in therapy, I learned that this elusive feeling was what I had been searching for during the first half of my life. Choosing inappropriate or unavailable partners was my way of proving how lovable I was. If I was able to get this person to love me, that meant I was a really good person and finally worthy of the love that I didn't feel as a child.

I always knew my mom loved me no matter what, and she was very good about showing it. But I don't think there was enough that my mom could do to make up for the lack of emotional and physical affection I didn't receive from my dad.

It is incredibly harmful for girls *and* boys to have their value based upon external factors like what they do (chores, behaviors, performing in school), how much they weigh or what they look like and how much others like them. These external motivators cause children—and caused me—to look outside of themselves for love and approval. My self-worth became dependent on how others responded to me and how happy I made them. Every aspect of my life became about pleasing others so I could, in turn, feel good about myself.

Conditional love makes a child feel like they inherently are not worthy of love because of who they are, but that they must "perform" or do things in order to gain the attention, admiration and love all humans desire (Clark, 2018; link: https://thriveglobal.com/stories/the-power-of-forgiveness-3/). Children in these situations become externally driven and lose their own innate ability to trust their own decision-making, and to value themselves. They allow others to exert authority over them, instead of it coming from within.

I became a "people pleaser" and based my self-worth on the responses I got from other people in positions of authority. I constantly sought approval from others and although on the outside that made me a compliant child who was obedient in school and with adults, the reasons behind these behaviors were not mentally or emotionally healthy in any way.

This learned behavior helped me be seen as a good student who didn't get out of line too often in school. I had friends, but these traits did not come from a place of confidence and self-worth, but instead from a place of fear that no one would like me if I didn't "do something" to make them like me. My lovability was based upon how I performed in school and at home, and it seemed like my home rating was never as high as my school's.

Learning early on that the expression of emotions resulted in disapproval, I sought to suppress my emotions at all cost and do whatever it took to keep these feelings at bay and my emotions in check. Now, I had lots of choices when it came to avoiding these feelings, so why did I choose food and not alcohol, drugs or sex?

Alcohol and drug abuse runs rampant in my family and extended family, and I think it is that truth that caused me not to turn to drugs or alcohol for comfort. My earliest memories of being with my mom's side of the family on Christmas Eve was of a dark, scary room filled with cigarette smoke, loud voices and boisterous relatives I didn't know and that scared me. I was a constant figure on my mom's hip anytime we went to that side of the family for Christmas. That environment felt out of control, and it frightened me, so maybe that's what saved me from turning to illegal drugs or going the underage-drinking route.

There were such rigid categorizations of right and wrong in my house that I knew I could never get away with drugs, alcohol, or sex... those would incur a wrath I might not survive, and food would be the easiest because it was most readily available.

Food became the vehicle to help me not only meet my neglected emotional needs, but it also was there to help me deal with my feelings of low self-worth, low self-esteem and lack of confidence. Food really was a friend and looking back now, I should have been way more appreciative of how much it supported me and got me through tough times. But I can now have a healthier relationship with food, see it for what it truly does for me and change my perspective on what our future relationship will look like.

Stop and Jot #5

This quick write is especially important, so please do not hold anything back. Let it all out onto the paper.

- *Did you feel you were given conditional or unconditional love in your childhood home?*

- *If you came from a home that was filled with unconditional love, have you ever been in a relationship in which you felt you had to act a certain way to receive your partner's love?*

- *What did that look like for you?*

- *How did it make you feel then?*

- *What about now?*

- *How do you think these feelings have impacted you and your use of food in dealing with emotions?*

Give yourself ten minutes to write and then put down your notebook and walk away. Do something that will make you feel good, like going outside and taking some deep breaths, playing with your pet, hugging your kids, taking a bath... anything non-food related that will help you feel cared for.

Come back to your notebook, pick up where you left off and give yourself ten more minutes to write. Please don't go back and read, because it may provoke you to edit what you stated and the raw, real emotions are what you finally need to get out. These notes are for you only, so please be brutally honest about what you felt, and how you still feel. This is all part of the process. Again, take a break and revisit the prompts one last time for another ten minutes until you get everything out you feel needs to be released.

Next, put your notebook and this book away until tomorrow. This will give you time to process what you just released through writing. Go about your life and do not dwell on what you wrote, but see it as released from your body, heart and spirit. Feel yourself as lighter, freer and without the restraints of non-expression you have felt for most of your life. Keep these writings safely in your notebook for use later on, but for now, just be proud of yourself for getting these thoughts and feeling out on paper.

It is important to remember that your experiences with emotional eating are personal and individual, so not everything is going to apply to your particular situation. If something doesn't apply to you or has not been an issue for you in your past, appreciate that and acknowledge the positives in your upbringing. Take whatever pieces apply to you and your situation and work through them.

Where To Now?

In these first two chapters, you have done some powerful work in addressing and acknowledging your issues with food. You have looked at the family dynamics in your childhood and how they impacted the development of your relationship with food. You've also had an opportunity to look back and see where specific things might have been done or said that prevented you from sharing how you felt or from expressing your emotions when you were young.

You might be wondering how all these things tie together, and what they have to do with your eating. In reality, they have everything to do with why you choose to eat when you do. It is these discovered factors that contribute to your ongoing feelings of reliance on food to get you through difficult situations.

Food has become a replacement, a distractor and a form of comfort for you during times of stress, anxiety or sadness.

In the next chapter, you are really going to nail down when the defining events happened in your childhood that prompted you to stop eating only when hungry, to use food as an elixir or a way of making yourself feel better when confronted with uncomfortable circumstances or situations.

Once you process that information, you will be able to move on to the most important step you can take...and that is letting go of these events, forgiving those involved and rewriting the story of your childhood to make it healthy, nurturing and loving.

Chapter 3
The Truth About Your Why

Newborn babies are amazingly healthy eaters. When they are hungry, they cry, and when they are full, they stop eating and usually fall asleep. Their little bodies are working so hard to grow and develop; naturally, they know when they need more sustenance to keep up with all their ever-changing needs for energy.

Some people move through their childhoods and into being an adult and never lose that instinctual ability to eat only when hungry, but for the majority of the population, that is not the case.

When does the shift happen? What happens to make us stop eating only when hungry and develop an unhealthy reliance on food to provide something other than nutrients?

A phenomenon called Eating in the Absence of Hunger (EAH) can develop in children as young as three years old and is the loss of the natural ability to self-regulate hunger. A 2018 study showed that feeding strategies used in the home have a significant impact on a child's relationship with food, and that these messages are both direct and passive in nature. The primary caregiver often delivers these messages to children without even being aware of it. When kids experience patterns of restrictive eating, as well as pressure to eat more than needed, these episodes contribute to children developing a negative relationship with food and making EAH a more regular occurrence (Castle, 2017; link: https://health.usnews.com/wellness/for-parents/articles/2017-07-05/why-do-kids-eat-when-theyre-not-hungry).

The passive experiences could be something as innocent as a mom discussing with her best friend how she needs to cut back on eating bread, within earshot of her daughter. The study indicated that young girls were more impacted by exposure to restrictive eating patterns than boys. Boys were more likely to experience direct messages about their caregiver's desire to have them eat more food than they needed. This can result in the loss of the natural mechanism that prevents overeating (Castle, 2017; link: https://health.usnews.com/wellness/for-parents/articles/2017-07-05/why-do-kids-eat-when-theyre-not-hungry).

It sounds so cliché and "therapy-like", but you must go back and examine where and when in your childhood your natural instinct to regulate your own hunger sensations was turned on its ear and you started eating for reasons other than hunger. As mentioned before, this is not about pointing fingers and blaming anyone, especially your parents, for the situation you find yourself in.

Parenting is the hardest job in the world, and there is no instruction manual as to how to raise a healthy, well-adjusted child. Truthfully, I don't think it is possible in today's society, but it is *essential* to remember that all parents do the best job they can to raise their kids based upon the information they have available from their own upbringing or education.

For many, this process is extremely painful and brings up many feelings of resentment, guilt, shame, etc., and if doing these types of exercises makes you uncomfortable, it is time to look at why you feel that way and address the situation. Otherwise, you are repeating the same pattern all over again. Uncomfortable feelings lead to diverting attention away by distracting with food and relying on its presence to comfort and soothe. In reality, that is something you should be doing through communication.

There are six circumstances that might have contributed to you losing your ability to naturally regulate your food consumption (Castle, 2017; link: https://health.usnews.com/wellness/for-parents/articles/2017-07-05/why-do-kids-eat-when-theyre-not-hungry). As you read each description, think about whether this might apply to your childhood, and if it is something that still might be impacting you.

1. **Lack of appetite awareness:** Members of "The Clean Plate Club" lose their sensation of appetite awareness because forcing a child to eat more than they need can override the appropriate appetite response. An example would be having a baby finish a bottle or eat an entire jar of baby food after they have indicated they are no longer hungry.

2. **High responsiveness to food:** When a child is in an environment in which accessibility to food is either excessive or limited, children can develop extreme reactions to food that place too much importance on it. Food needs to be

predictable and a normal part of daily living, not something that has too much importance placed on it.

3. **Impulsive around food:** A child with low inhibitory control may be impulsive in many situations, and food presents a special issue. When foods are denied or restricted, it makes them that much more appealing and may lead to behaviors that limit a child's ability to stop eating when satisfied.

4. **Self-soothing with food:** Encouraging a child to talk about their feelings instead of giving them food to make them feel better is essential in order to avoid developing the habit of soothing emotions with food. The earlier in life kids are taught to talk about their feelings instead of distracting themselves with an activity or substance, the healthier a child will be, both emotionally and physically.

5. **Boredom:** Eating because there is nothing else to do can quickly become a habit that a child turns to in order to avoid feelings of loneliness or boredom. It also sets up a child for mindless eating, when they become conditioned to eat

without any attention being given to their satisfaction or fullness in relationship to the food consumed. This can set up a habit of disconnection between the mind and body.

6. **Food restrictions:** When certain foods are "off limits" to kids, these foods become much more desirable and revered and can result in kids becoming obsessed with foods they are not allowed to consume. When they *do* have access to these foods, there is a greater likelihood they will overconsume due to feeling scarcity and a feeling these foods may never be available to them again. This can also result in the habit of sneaking food or eating in secret due to the forbidden nature placed upon these foods.

Did any of these circumstances resonate with you as a possible situation that might have been present in your childhood? Did you feel an emotional reaction as your read the descriptions, and what were those feelings all about?

Stop and Jot #6

In your journal, select each of the circumstances outlined above that you believe were a part of your childhood, and describe how you think they might have impacted your loss of the natural ability to self-regulate your food consumption. For each scenario, answer the following questions:

- *Do you remember having this type of situation occur in your early childhood? If the answer is no, move on to the next circumstance. If yes, explain the situations where it occurred.*

- *What were the specific conditions that resulted in this happening (if you can remember)?*

- *How did these episodes of eating make you feel both during and after they happened?*

- *How do you see this still playing out in your life today?*

A Personal Illustration

An example from my childhood would be my own high level of responsiveness to food. My extended family on my dad's side was very close and getting together for holidays was always something I looked forward to because of the array of incredible foods served at these events. My nona and my mom were incredible cooks, and as you recall, being from the South, food was a way of expressing love. The foods served at these get-togethers always surpassed my expectations, and I so clearly remember feeling like since we didn't get these foods too often that I had to eat as much as I could. I knew they were not a part of our regular diet, so I was not going to get to have these dishes again anytime soon, so I should eat as much as I could, even if that meant overeating.

The anticipation of these holiday meals was unusually high, and I can remember cutting back on my eating in the days that preceded them so I could justify to myself why it was okay to overindulge. It set up in my mind the thought that anytime there was a special meal or event, I had to eat as much as I could of these "special foods" because they would be going away, and I might not have them again for a very long time.

The feelings of almost desperation and panic at not getting to have these foods was evident, so I would always eat to the point of discomfort just to be able to be sure I got enough of the foods served.

It was not about the taste of the food (although the taste was amazing); it was the positive associations I had with these events and how much the food made me feel a part of things, like I fit in with my family. Everyone always over-indulged, and it was just what I did to feel connected to the other members of my family.

This presents itself in my life in a variety of ways. Any meal that I have outside of my home I view as "special" and "exclusive," so I go into these meals feeling like I better eat as much of these foods as I possibly can because I may never have them again. Inevitably, I developed the habit of overeating when at a restaurant or a friend's house because of this fear of scarcity, and as a result, would try to avoid these types of situations because my behavior would be so out of control.

I have learned to talk myself through the emotions that come up in these times and remind myself that all foods are always available to me. The fear that I won't have access to these foods again is not real, and I remind myself that I always have enough of what I need and that it won't be taken away from me.

Going through each of these scenarios and processing the emotions that are related to them is so important because it allows you to see how automatically and habitually these thought processes happen, and we don't even realize it. Awareness is the first step in changing a dysfunctional pattern and then learning a new way to respond that will serve you in a positive way.

So What Is This Really About?

If you only ate when you were hungry and stopped eating when you were full, you would not have an issue with your weight. It is clear that somewhere in your childhood you lost that ability, and food became about so much more than filling a physiological need.

Your weight issue is not about the foods you eat, but about the emotions associated with food that you developed in your childhood (Smith et al, 2018; link: https://www.helpguide.org/articles/diets/emotional-eating.htm/). Those emotions are uncomfortable, they are habitual, and they result in you eating for the wrong reasons.

Don't blame food... it is not the enemy. It is there is provide you energy and allow you to go through life doing the things you physically want to do. It is time to stop looking at food to solve our problems, and to start dealing with our issues head-on.

As examined in Chapter 2, if you were raised in an environment where expressing emotions was not permitted or encouraged, that not only is going to be something foreign to you and not your natural reaction, but it is also something that you might have few skills in executing appropriately.

It is time to rip off the Band-Aid and look at where this unhealthy dependence on food came from so it can be acknowledged, forgiven and let go. Creating a new reality for your childhood allows you to change your thought processes toward eating.

Food and the Addiction Process

Food, like alcohol, drugs, sex, and gambling, can be used like any of these more commonly known addictive substances to take you away from your reality and numb you to the uncomfortable or disturbing circumstances you would rather avoid. Addiction works exactly the same, whether ice cream or vodka, and the result can be just as devastating.

Addiction to any substance or process is defined as involvement with a substance (alcohol/drugs) or process (gambling/sex) that results in substantial harm to an individual, and this pattern is repeated even though the harm is acknowledged and recognized. Because the circumstance is pleasurable, or perceived as such, the behaviors continue (Horvath, Misra, Epner & Cooper, n.d; link: https://www.mentalhelp.net/articles/definition-of-addiction/).

There is very likely an emotional dependence on the substance or process that makes the user think they can't get by without it. They must have whatever it is that gets them through discomfort, and it is believed they need it more than they do (Melemis, 2018; link: https://www.addictionsandrecovery.org/what-is-addiction.htm).

Process addictions, which include eating, seek to find comfort and avoid feelings through the behavior of choice (Horvath et al., n.d; link:

https://www.mentalhelp.net/articles/definition-of-addiction/). The act of eating temporarily distracts the user from having to confront and deal with the emotions at hand. The food that is being consumed is not the problem; it is the thought processes and the resulting behaviors surrounding food that are the issue.

The brain can be trained to respond to certain foods and start to crave them in times of stress (Scalise, n.d; link: https://brainspeak.com/how-negative-self-talk-sabotages-your-health-happiness/). Now, if you were able to train your brain to crave broccoli during times of stress that would be fabulous, but that is not how the brain works. The pleasure center of the brain wants to be made happy, so it is going to crave high-fat, high-carb, sugar-filled foods to give the brain and body the rush of increased blood sugar it needs to create a euphoric feeling (Scalise, n.d; link: https://brainspeak.com/how-negative-self-talk-sabotages-your-health-happiness/).

The body and the mind can together create cravings that are so strong and powerful that they are challenging, if not almost impossible, to resist. Combine that with an inability to address and deal with challenging emotions, and you have the perfect storm for eating an excess of calories that will result in weight gain.

Identify Your Triggers

There are many situations, circumstances, emotions and foods that can cause an episode of emotional eating to occur. Before now, they may have seemed random and to have occurred without warning or reason, but as you are coming to realize, these circumstances are anything but random and occur as a result of situations in your past that cause these emotions or memories to come to the surface. Once at the surface, you have the opportunity to either face them and feel them or try to distract yourself and avoid them at all costs. Avoidance has resulted in eating excess calories and weight gain, but what if you were able to anticipate these triggers, try to avoid them, or if confronted you had a plan for how to address them? The feeling of empowerment and confidence would be amazing and could permeate all areas of your life, causing an increase in self-esteem and self-worth.

Researchers at PsychTests surveyed 438 identified emotional eaters and were able to establish the following as the nine most common eating triggers (Jerabek, n.d; link: http://consciouslivingtv.com/health/whats-eating-you.html):

1. **Lack of Intimacy**—Foods serve as the comfort yearned for from a partner, friend or family member. Even if a support system is in place, emotional eaters quite often feel lonely and food serves as a replacement for intimacy.

2. **Feelings of Shame**—If a transgression has occurred in the past, emotional eaters will continue to beat themselves up via food, even if they have been forgiven. The focus is on disappointments, regrets and what is wrong with themselves and their lives.

3. **Fear of Challenges**—The belief that failure is possible causes emotional eaters to avoid challenging situations and seek comfort and distraction through food.

4. **Fear of Judgment**—Emotional eaters have high expectations for their own body image and if they haven't reached it, they punish themselves. They fear rejection from others, so they do it to themselves before others have a chance.

5. **Conflict Avoidance**—Instead of expressing emotions and feelings, food is used to distract and comfort.

6. **Boredom**—Mindless eating is simpler and easier to do than an engaging activity, and fear of failure results in eating out of boredom.

7. **Self-Sabotaging Beliefs**—Limiting beliefs about their own abilities to make changes to their bodies and make wise food choices results in a lack of confidence or belief they can be successful. It is better to sabotage yourself and be in control of it, than to fail simply because you aren't good enough. Emotional eaters choose to be in control.

8. **Rebellion**—If foods during childhood were restricted or forbidden, or the household was very rigid with strict rules about everything, as an adult, an emotional eater may be seeking their own kind of freedom and liberation through food.

9. **Physical, Emotional or Sexual Abuse**—Trauma is a risk factor for disordered eating, and emotional eaters may seek to punish or shame themselves

through food as a way of inflicting pain, as if the abuse was somehow their fault.

Slowly re-examine this list and know that you may have a number of triggers depending on the environment you are in or the people you are around.

Stop and Jot #7

In your journal, label this entry, "What are my triggers?". Go through each of the questions below to determine what your personal triggers are in relationship to emotional eating. Use the list above as a guide and know that you may have multiple triggers. Once you identify what your triggers are, you are better able to objectively deal with them as they occur and come up with coping strategies to help you avoid eating in these circumstances.

- *Think back through the last few times you felt you were eating for emotional reasons instead of physical hunger. Recall the circumstances prior to eating... what happened prior to you starting to eat?*

- *What were your emotions in that moment?*

- *Is there a connection between these feelings and a childhood circumstance that brings up those emotions?*

Apply these questions to at least two situations in which you have found yourself eating for non-physical hunger reasons. Write as much as you can about how you were feeling in that moment and where in your childhood you think those emotions originated. Again, it is not about blaming anyone: It is acknowledgement of where these emotional reactions came from so you can choose to respond as an adult in a different way.

A Personal Illustration

Social situations have long been a trigger for my emotional eating, but the actual eating part rarely happened at the actual event. I maintained a good facade in front of my friends but once I was able to escape these situations, once I got home, I found myself eating uncontrollably.

For approximately 13 of my 17 years as a middle school teacher I chaired the social committee, and I was in charge of organizing both the holiday party and end-of-the-year party. The last holiday party I helped with stands out in my mind as a perfect example of how social situations and my feelings of not "fitting in" or not being "good enough" caused me to resort to secret eating to help me through a difficult situation.

The party was at our Spanish teacher's house, and I arrived early with the other members of the social committee to get things set up. The party started and things were progressing along smoothly... nothing occurred that should have set me off but as people arrived and I again felt that stab of being a "single" at an event where most people brought their spouse or significant other, I started to feel the anxiety build, and I knew I needed to get myself out of the situation.

Fortunately, there were enough people at the party that I was able to slip away undetected, but not without packing up a plateful of desserts (that I had made for the party) and return to my quiet home. It took no more than five minutes for the plateful of desserts to be wiped out, but the eating did not stop there. I rummaged through my pantry and although I chose not to keep lots of food in my house, I ate whatever I could find to help rid me of the feelings of loneliness and isolation I felt. Not only was I upset that AGAIN I had to attend an event without a partner/husband/boyfriend, but I had left one uncomfortable situation (the party) to put myself in an equally upsetting situation (all alone at home while others were still having fun at the party).

None of this had been done *to* me... this was all self-imposed, and I had created the circumstances myself, but that didn't matter. The feelings were still there and they were still "treated" with a plateful of food that I wasn't hungry for and felt horrible about eating afterward.

Stop and Jot #8

Label this journal entry, "Trigger, Response, and Source" and go back to your list from Chapter 1 called "Emotional Eating Encounters." You wrote down and grouped together circumstances where emotional eating was more likely to take place. You have learned so much over the course of the first three chapters and you now have a handle on what types of things set you up for emotional eating.

- *You are now going to take each of the "encounters" you listed and write down:*

    1. *The trigger that set off the situation*

    2. *What your emotional response was (anger, sadness, fear, boredom)*

    3. *Where you think this reaction came from in your childhood.*

This is a very important exercise, so please take your time and be as thorough as possible in your responses. This will greatly help you in the next chapter as we look to rewrite the childhood circumstances that have resulted in the need to emotionally eat to avoid your emotions and dysfunctional beliefs.

Chapter 4
I Know Where It Came From, But Now What?

Accept. Forgive. Rewrite.

These are the themes for this chapter, and they will change your life moving forward IF you can embrace them.

Acceptance is "a person's assent to the reality of a situation" (Fish, 2014, p.4; link: https://www.psychologytoday.com/us/blog/looking-in-the-cultural-mirror/201402/tolerance-acceptance-understanding). In the case of your childhood and circumstances that might be viewed as dysfunctional, acceptance of how you were raised and the events that occurred is the first step in being able to move past them. Acceptance does not mean that you give consent to what happened, it merely means that you choose to see the reality of the situation. You might not like it, but you can accept that it did occur, whatever the reason.

Forgiveness is a whole other ball of yarn. Psychologists define forgiveness as "...*a conscious, deliberate decision to release feelings of resentment or vengeance toward a person or group who has harmed you, regardless of whether they actually deserve your* **forgiveness....Forgiveness** *does not mean forgetting, nor does it mean condoning or excusing offenses*" (Clark, 2018, p.2-3; link: https://thriveglobal.com/stories/the-power-of-forgiveness-3/). This feels good as an explanation because it allows for a person to let go of the feelings they have inside and to free themselves of any bad energy while still being able to acknowledge they do not think whatever occurred was permissible or tolerable. When you forgive, you don't do it for the person who did the act... you forgive in order to free yourself from any negative energy.

And lastly, the act of rewriting, and in our case of rewriting your childhood stories to make them work for you as an adult, is the most liberating, empowering and courageous thing you can do for yourself. You do not have to be a victim of your past... you can be the creator of your glorious future merely by changing your perspective and viewpoint of a certain situation.

Now, I know the two on the end are much easier to digest than the loaded word in the middle, but you will take baby steps to make that word palatable and provide you with peace and serenity in your relationship with food, and with others in your life, like you might have never known before.

When we deny the story, it defines us. When we own the story, we can write a brave new ending. ~Brene Brown

As you start the process of accepting, forgiving and rewriting your story, you need to be sure you are open to the emotions and feelings that inevitably will arise as you dig deep into your past. Feelings of shame, disappointment, anger and resentment can come to the surface and although you can never anticipate or guarantee how a situation is going to unfold, you need to be aware that these circumstances may arise and be prepared to address them as they do.

The Role of Limiting Beliefs

We all have thoughts in our heads that are constantly either building us up or tearing us down, and limiting beliefs are especially effective at the latter. They are beliefs you have about yourself that were put upon you at some point in your life, most often during childhood. You came to believe they were true, and as a result, these beliefs have prevented you from doing many of the things you have wanted to do, or fully being the person you want to be (James, 2013; link: https://www.psychologytoday.com/us/blog/focus-forgiveness/201311/4-steps-release-limiting-beliefs-learned-childhood).

As an emotional eater, you have many beliefs about yourself and your body that have greatly impacted the choices you have made and the thoughts you have had about yourself. An example of a limiting belief is, "I'm big-boned and that is why I am overweight," or "I look at food and I gain weight." Somewhere along the line, these beliefs were given to you and you believed them, hook, line, and sinker. But the fact is they are what they say they are—*beliefs,* not truths—and every moment of every day, you have the opportunity to choose to buy into them or deny their existence.

Now, that's so much easier said than done because the reality is, these beliefs have been ingrained into your subconscious and your mind automatically goes to the thoughts that are most automatic, whether they serve you positively or not. It is your job, as an adult, to realize when a belief is not serving you in a positive way and seek to change that belief into something that works in your favor.

But how do you do that? The following process is based on the work of Dr. Matt James, who specializes in Neuro-Linguistic Programming and chronicled these steps as a guest contributor for Psychology Today in 2013.

Stop and Jot #9

Label your journal entry, "Letting Go of Limiting Beliefs."

Steps to process and release limiting beliefs:

Step 1: Write down all limiting beliefs you have about yourself in relationship to your weight and your body. Example—"I lose weight, but I always gain it back," or "losing weight is so hard."

Stop and Jot #9 *(Continued)*

Step 2: Embrace that these thoughts are beliefs, NOT truths. Your mind will fight you on this, but you must tell yourself and believe that these beliefs were given to you but are not who you are.

Step 3: Rephrase each belief to reflect what you want. Example—"I lose weight and keep it off because I love myself so much," or "Losing weight comes easy to me because I value my health."

Step 4: Take action as if your belief is true. Example—What action would a person take who loses weight because they love themselves? They would commit to exercise for 30 minutes, five days a week and would make it happen.

For each new belief, list two actions you will take to make it a truth in your life.

Here are some questions to ask yourself before moving forward in the process:

- Am I ready to take a look at the limiting beliefs that were put upon me in my childhood without blaming or finger-pointing?

- Can I look at these situations and accept that anger, resentment and disappointment might rise up in me?

- Am I prepared to address these emotions in a healthy (non-food) way so they can be processed but don't result in more stress on me?

- Can I look at my caregivers in an empathetic way and realize they were only doing their best with the knowledge they had?

- Can I forgive them, accept responsibility for being an adult and make the changes I need to make so my life can be the best it can be?

I have said this before, but it bears repeating: This book is not about blaming your parents or caregivers for your issues with food, or anything else in your life. It is about accepting what transpired in your childhood that makes you who you are, both the good and the not-so good, and making a decision, as an adult, how you want to proceed in your life given those circumstances.

All parents do the best they can to raise their children given their own upbringing, experiences and knowledge. I don't think any parent thinks to themselves, "Boy, if I could really jack my kid up and give them all kinds of personal issues, I'd do it in a heartbeat." I believe people do not have ill intent for others but are acting out of what they have inside their hearts based upon how they were treated or taught things.

Everyone does the best they can do.

Accept and Forgive

You have identified events in your childhood that you believe may have contributed to your dysfunctional relationship with food. You have also been able to pinpoint certain situations or circumstances that are triggers for you and cause you to want to eat food instead of deal with how you are feeling, and you know that these originated in your childhood.

It is now time to take each of these situations and accept that this is what happened, and it was through no fault of your own. You didn't "do" anything wrong, these were just the cards you were dealt in this area of your life and what happened is what happened. End of story.

The sooner you can accept that this is what happened, the easier it will be to move on to the next step, which is forgiveness. This step might not be so easy, but it is *so* vital, and you must remember that you are not forgiving the other person to make them feel better; you are doing it to allow yourself to be free from the chains of anger, resentment and blame.

I love the parts of the definition of forgiveness that mentions that you should forgive, "regardless of whether they actually deserve your **forgiveness**," and "nor does it mean condoning or excusing offenses." This allows you to release any feelings of hostility you might be harboring while not saying that the behavior is permissible.

I had learned in my first round of therapy in my mid-20s that I needed to forgive my dad for the fact that I never felt that he loved me because he never said the words to me. I held on to this for years, and it greatly impacted my ability to allow people to be close to me because I didn't allow myself to believe that anyone would ever love me. Why should I think that if my own father couldn't love me?

I thought I had let it go at that time, but I don't think I really bought into the whole belief that "parents do their best based upon what they were taught and how they were treated as kids." It wasn't until about five years ago that I was finally able to fully forgive my dad for what I perceived as the reasons why I had an eating disorder and why I couldn't have a normal relationship with food.

It was Thanksgiving and my then 18-year-old nephew, Ryan, was given an assignment to interview one of his grandparents about their upbringing and life, and so he chose to interview his Poppy, my dad. Ryan had a series of questions to ask my dad, and the entire family sat around and listened as my dad told the story of his early life.

He told about how at five years old, he had fallen out of the backseat of his mom's car going 35 miles per hour and was hospitalized for more than a week, his parents not knowing if he would survive. How he had to do the dishes every night for more than two years because his older sister was confined to her bed in a full-body cast after having had 18 surgeries to correct a deformed leg. And finally, he talked about the incredibly high expectations that were placed on my him as a very talented young athlete (my dad was drafted by the Detroit Tigers as a pitcher right out of high school) and how his father, my Popa, never told him how proud he was of his accomplishments.

As my dad was talking, he became overcome with emotions, started to cry and had to excuse himself because he couldn't continue to talk about his own childhood and the things he had been through. It was in that moment that I realized how broken my own dad was, and that he never meant to do anything that would end up hurting me... he just did the best he could. He was only being the parent that he had had modeled for him.

Talk about a liberating moment! I was able to release the resentment I had carried around for years and was finally able to see my dad in a totally different way. Our relationship was forever altered, and my dad and I are closer now than we have ever been.

I have been blessed to be able to go through the process I am about to outline for you with my dad (without him knowing it, of course), and have released the weight of anger and blame I placed on him for so many years about where my life was. It had become very easy to pile all of my disappointments onto him and how he raised me, because then I did not have to take responsibility for my life. It let me off the hook in that moment, and it felt good to feel like the victim, but being in "victim mode" will paralyze your growth if you allow it to. You have a built-in scapegoat to blame all your shortcomings on instead of making decisions and changes to better your situation. It can become a very safe place, but please, don't let it be.

You have picked up this book to help you with your relationship with food and in turn, it will help you with your relationship with others in your life, including yourself, if you allow it.

Stop and Jot #10

Label this entry, "Accept and Forgive." In your journal, list each of the instances from your childhood you feel contributed to your dysfunctional relationship with food, who provided you with this limiting belief and how it made you feel at that time.

Stop and Jot #10 (Continued)

Here is an example:

- *I was restricted from having certain foods like Pepsi, dry-roasted peanuts and Vitamin D milk by my dad, and it sent the message to me that I was fat and not worthy of eating these foods. It created the belief that there were "good" foods and "bad" foods, and that I was not allowed to eat the bad foods.*

Now, I want you to take that instance and accept and forgive that this situation was a part of your upbringing and let it go. If you feel you might even know why this situation occurred, you can include that as well. Here is my example:

- *I accept that my dad set up a system in our house that certain foods were off-limits to everyone but him, and this resulted in me believing I was fat. Clearly, this is something he learned from his own dad, and he thought it was the right thing to do to help his kids and wife avoid a weight problem.*

He had no idea it would do the opposite, and I forgive him for that. I let this go, and it is no longer a part of my relationship with food.

You may need to break this activity up into multiple stop-and-jots since it might get a bit overwhelming and emotional for you. Please take care of yourself and do it in a way that shows self-care and love.

Rewriting Your Food Story

The final step in this process is taking your beliefs about your relationship with food and rewriting them to reflect what you want them to be. Your mind is incredibly powerful and when you realize that as an adult, you have the choice to decide what kinds of thought patterns you adopt and embrace. You want to change those patterns of thinking to reinforce the changes you want to occur.

Now, how do you do that when it isn't true in the present moment? Hold on to your panties; I am about to get scientific on you.

We become what we repeatedly think.

This statement is absolutely true, and it is based on scientific facts. Patterns of thinking, both positive and negative, become etched into the nerve pathways in your brain over time, and the reactions the body and mind have to these repeated patterns becomes as automatic as driving a car. Every moment of every day, you have the choice to create positive thought patterns within your brain and significantly improve the quality of your life... or you can do the opposite.

The prefrontal cortex (the part of your brain responsible for setting goals and executing them) and the amygdala (the fear-based emotion-control center) can both be rewired over time so the cortex is able to stop the pathway of negative thoughts that can occur automatically and have the amygdala be bypassed so the emotion center of the brain does not become involved.

You are not ever able to completely rid yourself of negative thoughts or fears; it is part of our survival mechanism to keep us safe from dangerous situations. But, in learning to make peace with the negative thoughts in your head and accepting that they are a part of life, you can take away their power and start the rewiring process mentioned above.

The bottom line is this: You have control of your response to the thoughts in your head and you can either be in control of them or let them control you.

You want to be in control, and you will be.

This process really is surprisingly simple, but it does require persistence, patience, resilience and lots and lots of compassion and understanding. And it is all directed at you.

You have accepted and forgiven those responsible for creating the beliefs about food that have not been serving you, and now, you need to rewrite your story about food so it serves you every day. By writing and saying these statements, you are doing the work of rewiring your brain to accept that this is in fact your new way of thinking, and it will become as automatic as brushing your teeth in the morning.

Stop and Jot #11

Label this entry, "Rewriting Your Food Story."

Think about all the things you have discovered thus far about your relationship with food, and what your reactions are to food that have not been working for you. Make a list of them now. Think about all your limiting beliefs, even the ones that might not be directly related to food but that impact your self-esteem and confidence.

Example:

- *I eat mindlessly at night because I am lonely.*

- *I was denied fattening foods as a child.*

- *I believed I was fat because I was not allowed to eat certain foods.*

- *I was abandoned by my sister when I was moved to the room downstairs next to my parents' room.*

- *I eat when I am not hungry to distract me from what is really bothering me.*

- *I do not say what I think and feel because I am afraid of people not liking me.*

For each one of the statements made, rewrite that belief into a positive statement, or change it to reflect how you want your relationship with food to be:

Example:

- *When alone at night, I do things that make me feel happy and loved.*

- *I have access to any foods I want to eat, and nothing is off-limits.*

- *I love my body for all it does for me every day.*

- *I know my parents were only trying to keep me safe when they separated me from my sister; it taught me to be strong and that I could get by on my own.*

- *I only eat when I am hungry, and I stop when I am full.*

- *I speak my mind and my feelings, especially if I am upset with someone.*

This is THE MOST IMPORTANT writing assignment in this process, so please be as thorough as you can and write down as many of your limiting beliefs and also be thoughtful in your rewriting of the belief. It is this step, this reworking of the neural pathways, that will change your thought processes, and in turn, change your reactions to situations involving food. Be exhaustive, honest and vulnerable. Get everything out in your journal. I advise that you break this writing assignment into a few sessions to give yourself a chance to see how you feel and process those emotions.

Congratulations on some of the most powerful and life-changing work you can do for yourself. The very exciting aspect of this process is that you can apply it to any area of your life you are struggling to get a handle on. Changing the stories and tapes of how you feel about yourself and who you are is a challenging process and for many; it can be too difficult to confront. Please be incredibly proud of yourself for the deep work you have completed, and how you have chosen to move your life in a positive direction and be the creator of your destiny.

Chapter 5
So... the Problem's Gone, Right?

Oh, how I wish that were true.

I would so love to tell you that once you have gone through the steps of recognizing your limiting beliefs about eating, discovered where they came from, accepted that it happened, forgave those involved and then rewrote your story, that everything in your life would be unicorns and rainbows.

Sadly, that would be a lie, and I am not a liar.

As I told you earlier, I *so* believed that my food issues would be something that, if I worked hard enough, tried my best and was a good enough person, would go away and I would never have to think about food, my weight or what I looked like ever again.

Sadly, Dorothy, you're not in Kansas anymore, and that just isn't ever going to happen.

Like any other kind of addiction, food issues do not go away; instead, you learn to manage your reactions and responses to them. You and I will always be works in progress, and to me, that is exactly as it should be.

To move forward and take what you have learned in the previous chapters and apply it to your specific circumstances, you must also go into your future with a plan for how you are going to address the inevitable emotional situation when it arises and food starts calling your name.

In the words of my very wise personal coach, Dave Smith, "What gets planned is what gets done." You can think about things you want to have happen, but until you come up with a formulated plan for accomplishing something, it is merely just a *thought* and not an *action*. Make a plan on paper and things get done.

I am going to break up the planning for dealing with feelings of emotional eating in three phases: *The Big Picture, Planning for Challenges, and In the Moment.* Each phase will address how to incorporate certain habits, strategies and routines into your life to better prepare you for times of challenge and stress. As I said earlier, life isn't suddenly going to be rainbows and unicorns. The inevitable crisis will arise, and you will be faced with the choice to give in to emotional eating. The better equipped you are to deal with these situations, the more confident and powerful you will be.

So let's take each phase and break down what things you can do to fortify your resolve to conquer the demon of emotional eating each time it rears its ugly head.

The Big Picture

The strategies and suggestions presented are meant to be large, overarching, life-changing tools that if incorporated into your life will not only improve the quality of your relationships with others but also your ability to more appropriately handle your relationship with food. These are "big picture" items because they work on your life at a level that is impactful in very specific ways but also in the overall grand scheme of things.

Changing Thoughts

Managing your emotional responses to various situations is vital in your learning to deal with, and work through, episodes of emotional eating. These ten tips, based on the 2014 article entitled, "Conquer Emotional Eating with These 12 Weird Tricks", will help you make emotional eating a thing of the past.

1. **Change the Words You Say to Yourself**—Instead of "...when I eat healthy, I feel deprived and pissed off," say, "I'm proud of myself for loving myself so much that I make healthy choices." Creating positive emotions from your thoughts is a trait that is learned and mastered, but unfortunately not over-night. It takes patience to learn how to do this and then maintain it. Cognitive Behavior Therapy is the technique most often used in circumstances like this, and it changes the brain's interpretation of situations and creates positive emotions.

2. **Create a New Rewards System**—Reward yourself in non-food ways that will make you happy: go for a walk, watch a show you love on Netflix, buy yourself

something special or give yourself the spa treatment you've always wanted. It is so important to retrain your brain to want rewards that do not involve food.

3. **Treat Yourself as You Would a Child**—You would speak to a loved child with kindness and sensitivity, and that is exactly how you should speak to yourself. Protect your emotional self because when it feels safe, strong and protected, emotional eating will no longer need to be a reaction because its emotional needs are being taken care of.

4. **Commit to Yourself**—Stick to your goals, keep the promises you make to yourself and commit daily to self-care: This will create a feeling of self-motivation.

5. **Keep Junk Food Out of the House**— Show yourself love and commitment by not having fat-filled snacks around to tempt you.

6. **Create a New Identity Through Visualizations**—Visualize yourself with all the traits you expect to have once the program is completed. Adopting a new,

healthier, more-empowered identity will help dissipate emotional eating; you will not need it as a crutch any longer.

7. **Reduce Your Stress**—Stress causes all kinds of chemical reactions in the body the most critical of which is an increase in the production of cortisol (a hormone that contributes to belly fat retention and weight gain). Incorporate mindfulness, meditation, yoga or just relaxing activities into your daily routine.

8. **Breathe**—Just simple breath will relax you and clear your mind. Taking three slow, deep breaths with your hand on your belly, called deep-belly breathing, allows the urge to eat to pass.

9. **Make it a Choice**—Create a pro/con list for emotional eating and focus on your desire to get control over your eating. Realize it is a choice: You are in control and have the power to choose to eat or not. A happier life is within your power.

10. **Change What You Value**—Decide to place top priority on your health and not on instant gratification. Value the long-

term goal and not what is going to make you feel good in the moment.

Scientific research shows the ability of the brain to change its chemical makeup through the thoughts you think about yourself. If hormones and neurotransmitters in the brain are out of balance, research shows that through affirmations and positive self-talk, these chemicals can be altered and can be used as tools to maintain a healthy mind, body and spirit (Talmay, 2014; link: https://www.huffington post.com/orion-talmay/conquer-emotional-eating-with-these-12-weird-tricks_b_5471268.html).

You have the means to harness the power of the mind-body connection to improve your health on all levels, and positive thinking and self-talk is the way to making that happen.

Meditation

Being anywhere but in the present moment is a hallmark of an episode of emotional eating. "Zoning out" while eating, often times not even being aware of what or how much you have eaten, is the end game you are looking to avoid.

You want to be removed from an uncomfortable, difficult situation, and food is the vehicle to take you there. Unfortunately, as good as it seems in the moment, that is the danger of these episodes. You become so removed and numbed that before you know it, physical damage from the overconsumption of high-fat junk foods has occurred, and it is too late to turn back.

Being present, in the moment and in touch with your body are skills that do not come naturally to most people; they need to be acquired and practiced. Developing a daily practice of meditation helps you connect with your body and yourself, so you can authentically feel your emotions and process them in a healthy way. This allows for you to take care of yourself in any given circumstance.

But how does meditation do that? In regard to emotional eating, practicing daily meditation helps in a variety of ways:

- It allows you to be in touch with your body so you can clue into feeling of emotional vs. physical hunger and allows you to learn how to use food for health and hunger.

- Stillness teaches you how to cultivate inner peace and provides you with a way to drop into that peace-filled state when things get crazy. This is life-changing. You will learn that you don't have to turn to emotional eating to cope with life's stresses and discomfort.

- Breath work associated with meditation will provide you with a built-in way of changing your state of being. In reality, when you binge eat, that is what you desire. Breath work will take the place of that.

- Meditation enables you to feel your emotions, sit with them and be okay in the process. This makes emotional eating unnecessary.

If you are anything like me, the idea of starting to meditate sounds really good but the actual sitting down and doing it is a whole other ball of wax. I know for me it was not so much finding the time but a fear I wouldn't do it correctly. From there, I would become frustrated and not want to continue to try.

In all honesty, meditation is not something you see results from right away. It takes time and patience, and those are not things I have a lot of. I want instant results, and that just doesn't happen with meditation.

There are many apps on the market that can assist you in understanding and adopting a meditation practice into your daily life. The one I have used is "Calm." It has a seven-day introductory series for beginners, and it not only walks you through guided meditations, but it also explains the concepts and reasoning behind meditation. For those of us who need to really think through why we are doing something, it is extremely helpful.

Yoga

Another strategy that will help you be more present in both mind and body is to begin a yoga practice. Regardless of what style of yoga you choose, yoga will help you develop a sense of calm and centeredness through postures, breathing, relaxation and mindfulness.

Yoga creates contentment through deep, smooth belly breathing that will leave you blissful and balanced. This will help during times of stress, grief and sadness. It teaches self-compassion and body acceptance and allows you to recognize that everyone is human and each person experiences difficult emotions. Yogis are taught to "be" with their emotions, both good and challenging, and are provided skills to face these emotions and not turn to food as an escape. Present-moment, in-your-body experiences are emphasized in yoga and strategies to keep yourself from acting mindlessly, whether related to food or not, are practiced in each session (Scriven,2017; link: https://www.doyouyoga.com/how-to-prevent-emotional-eating-using-yoga-57087/). A 12-week research study was done with obese women that included a weekly yoga class and a daily 30-minute home practice that provided the participants with yoga postures, calming breathing, relaxation techniques and a guided meditation. Results from the study showed that women reported less binge eating, higher self-esteem, more positive body image and a decrease in BMI (body mass index) and hip-to-waist ratio (Ross, Brooks, & Wallen, 2016; link: https://www.hindawi.com/journals/ecam/2016/2914745/).

Affirmations

Self-affirmations are statements you make about yourself in order to make your beliefs or thoughts about yourself more positive. Affirmations help to make you feel worthy of all the good things coming into your life as well as show compassion for self. Research has shown that your mind is your most powerful agent for change, and when thoughts are directed in a positive way toward yourself, only good things can come from it (Scalise, 2018; link: https://brainspeak.com/how-negative-self-talk-sabotages-your-health-happiness).

Affirmations act as motivation, because when you feel good about yourself, you are more likely to take action to make your life better. When done regularly, they can have an overall positive impact on your life because they eliminate the negative thoughts and feelings many people get wrapped up in when life is challenging (Scalise, 2018; link: https://brainspeak.com/how-negative-self-talk-sabotages-your-health-happiness). Positive thoughts attract more of the same, so affirmations bring many good things into your life and can positively impact the lives of others with whom you interact.

In relation to emotional eating, reinforcing new habits and beliefs about yourself and your ability to manage your eating will tremendously improve your ability to handle situations during which emotional eating may occur. Examples of food-related affirmations are:

- "I eat when I am hungry and stop when I am full."

- "I eat in proper portions."

- "I make wise food choices."

- "Eating healthy comes naturally to me."

- "Healthy, nutritious food is what I crave."

These types of positive statements about yourself and your beliefs are tremendously helpful in changing limiting beliefs you may have had, and create a more uplifting and empowering environment for you to thrive in.

There are many ways you can create and incorporate affirmations into your life. A number of websites provide affirmations to help improve any aspect of your life, from losing weight to making sales, quitting smoking and calming anxiety. All you need to do is select which ones resonate with you and start using them.

You can also write your own that are specific to your circumstances, but there are a couple of rules to follow to make sure they are successful. First, you must always write them in the present tense as if they are true in the present moment. Even if that feels strange, it trains the mind to believe the affirmations are already a fact. Next, they must be written in a positive way because our brains do not process negative. For example, instead of "I will not eat after 7 p.m.," say "I stop eating at 7 p.m." The mind doesn't recognize the "not," so it will get rid of it. Your affirmation is then doing the opposite by reinforcing, "I eat after 7 p.m." You must be sure to say your affirmation in the correct way to get the results you desire.

Lastly, in whatever way you desire, affirmations must be repeated in order to be effective. The more you repeat the same affirmation, the more your unconscious mind begins to believe it. By continually subjecting our mind to positive thoughts, we are actively changing how the brain functions. Over time, we are training our brains to think more positively through self-affirmations.

There are several ways to repeat your affirmations and make them more effective.

There are apps like *Think It Up* that allow you to record your voice saying your affirmations to listen to daily. You can also write them out every morning or night (or both) in a journal or say them out loud to yourself as well. I have even seen people write them on index cards and strategically place them around their house in order to find them at random times throughout the day. You can determine what style works for you and what measure of accountability you need to make them the most beneficial.

These recommended strategies and tips will improve anyone's life, whether or not they have an issue with emotional eating and will establish a foundation of positivity that will carry throughout all aspects of life. Your job, relationships, physical health, mental health and spirituality will be impacted in an incredibly positive way when these tools are committed to and included in a daily routine.

Planning for Food Challenges

The following suggestions are based upon the belief that "what gets planned is what gets done," meaning that if you have a plan in place for difficult situations when they pop up, you will be better equipped to address them mentally and spiritually. This will continue to reinforce the power of your positive beliefs about yourself and the good that is in your life.

Food Journaling

I will be honest, after 20-plus years of writing down every morsel of food that went into my mouth and giving it an approximate calorie count, I was hesitant to include food journaling as a suggestion to help with emotional eating. I truly believe the obsession I had with writing down everything I ate contributed to my issues, so it made me pause when I researched about this being a helpful strategy.

What I happily came to realize is, like anything else in life, it is all about your perspective and how you choose to interpret a situation. In this case, how I suggest you use a food journal is completely different and helpful in dealing with your food issues.

For emotional eating, your food journal is meant to be more of a feelings journal. I do not want you to list any foods you eat and write down a calorie count. Instead, I suggest that you note how you physically felt before you ate (were you truly hungry?), how you emotionally felt before you ate, if you were able to stop eating once you became satisfied and if there were any feelings of regret or guilt afterward.

This is the kind of information needed in order for you to then be able to analyze why the circumstance came up, what decision you made and how you felt about it afterwards. It also allows you to be able to take these situations and break them down, as we did in Chapter 4, to determine where they originated and how you can change your viewpoint. When going through the process from Chapter 4 of acceptance, forgiveness and rewriting, this information will prove to be quite helpful. In reality, as time goes on, you may uncover more issues related to food—ones that were there all along but that you missed the first time you went through this process—so having kept a record can be helpful.

Please know that I am not saying that you must keep a food journal for the rest of your life... oh, heck no... but I do think that when you are feeling challenged by your emotions and find yourself falling into old habits of using food to soothe emotions, this is an effective and reliable strategy to get you back on track and feeling in control of food.

Self-Care Plan

The most important thing you can do for yourself is the thing most of us rarely do. Self-care is far and away the most important strategy you can use to reduce the number of emotional eating episodes, because when we feel emotionally "fed," we have no need to look to food to fill our heart and soul with all that we think we are missing.

Always remember, more than anything else, that you are ENOUGH, as you are right now, reading this book. Even though you might feel like a hot mess, you are good enough and worthy of all the things you desire in your life without having to "do" anything to earn those things.

What does that look like, and how do you make the time for self-care?

Taking care of your needs means something different to each person. Many women spend most of their lives caring for everyone else yet have no idea what makes *them* feel happy or cared about. Does that sound like you? It is time to figure out what you can do to take care of yourself and give yourself the love and nurturing you need.

Stop and Jot #12

In your journal, label your entry, "My Self-Care" and make a list of at least ten things you can do for yourself to help you feel loved, cherished and cared for. Ask yourself these questions to help you come up with your list:

- *What is something that makes me feel special that only benefits me?*

- *Is there something I have not been doing that I know would put a smile on my face (that is not food-related)?*

- *What activity fills my heart with joy and happiness?*

Everyone's list will be different, but these pleasurable experiences will replace the "feel-good" feelings you get from food but will serve you in a positive way. Examples of self-care activities could be wearing soft clothes and fabrics that feel good against your skin, taking a bubble bath, buying yourself flowers, reading a favorite book in a quiet place in your home that is just for you or giving yourself a foot massage with essential oils or your favorite lotion. Have fun creating your list and be sure you make these things easily accessible so you can do this for yourself without much effort.

Now that you have created your personalized list of self-care actions, you need to incorporate it into your daily routine. It should become as automatic as brushing your teeth or making your bed in the morning.

I call this "Me Time", and the name comes from the work of Dr. Rangan Chatterjee, a primary care doctor and the star of the BBC series *Doctor in the House,* and it is far and away the most important thing anyone with emotional eating issues can do to help themselves get a better handle on the issue. I am about to suggest something so outrageous that I feel reasonably confident you are going balk at this initially and come up with five reasons why this absolutely can't happen. I understand your feelings of hesitation, but I am also going to show you how this not only is going to help you with your eating, but also in your goal to get to a healthy weight.

I want you to schedule 15 minutes of "Me Time" into your day, as if it were a doctor's appointment or a vital meeting at work and is not something that can be ignored. This time is going to do many things for you, the most important being helping you feel valued and cared for, so you don't have to then turn to food to feel taken care of. And secondly, it can definitely benefit any efforts you are making to lose weight because taking care of yourself has been shown to reduce stress and the stress in your life might be causing you to not be able to lose weight.

Dr.Chatterjee has been incorporating stress-reduction strategies into his practice to help patients improve their overall health and lose excess weight. He had a client who was frustrated because she was not losing weight despite incorporating all of Dr. Chatterjee's suggestions and doing everything correctly. She was about to give up when the doctor decided to give her a new strategy to try. He really felt that her problem was more stress-related and that she was producing too much cortisol, so he gave her a new "prescription,"

She was required to meditate for five minutes in the morning, and then at night give herself 15 minutes of relaxation time, or "Me Time," to help reduce her incredibly high levels of the stress hormone cortisol. She did this for four weeks and when she returned to see the doctor, she had lost 16 pounds without making any changes to her diet and exercise regimen.

I am not saying you'll lose 16 pounds in a month taking some "Me Time" every day, but I will tell you that numerous studies have shown the positive health benefits of reducing your stress through self-care. In your case, the positive result will be you feeling more fulfilled and valued, and that in turn will reduce the likelihood of your emotional eating to avoid negative feelings. If that is curtailed, weight loss is much more likely to occur.

In the Moment

The last area to examine as you prepare to live your life while managing your emotional eating is what I like to call "In the Moment". This is the time when you are in the trenches, emotions are flying, you are doing the "should I eat it or should I do something else" dance and you need to be as prepared as you can be to respond to what you are truly hungry for and not use food as a Band-Aid.

View the following as your "Emergency Kit" to get you out of the intense feelings that precede an emotional eating episode and safely move you to the other side of those emotions:

1. **Be Present and "Take 5"**—When you feel the urge to eat, stop and take five seconds to ask yourself these questions:

   - How is my stomach feeling?

   - Do I physically NEED to eat something?

   - What emotions am I feeling right now?

   - Will eating resolve the feelings I am having?

   By stopping and asking yourself these questions, you will become present in the moment and be able to make a decision about whether your desire to eat is physical or emotional. If it's physical, eat something nutritious; if emotional, refer to your list of self-care options and select one that will "feed" you in that moment (Smith et al, 2018; link: https://www.helpguide.org/articles/diets/emotional-eating.htm/).

2. **Remember Your Why**—You have a reason for feeling it was time to address your issues with emotional eating. That reason—your *why*—must be powerful enough to get you through hard times. Make a list of why dealing with your food issues is important, and then break it down even more. For each item listed, ask why, and answer it. Then, ask why again at least six or seven times until you get to the real reasons you want to address your eating issues. During challenging times, you must remember what those reasons are and let them be your motivation for not falling into the emotional eating trap.

3. **Keep Your Eyes on the Prize**—The outcome you want to see as a result of managing your food issues must stay at the forefront of your mind in order to be another motivating factor that keeps you from eating when not hungry. Creating a vision board of images you would like to have once you have a handle on your emotional eating can go a long way towards helping you stay the course. Using images from magazines, the Internet or old photos, create a collage of words and images that will remind you,

and the universe, what you would like to come into your life. When you send out positive messages, the universe listens and responds accordingly, bringing you what you ask for.

4. **Take Three Deep Breaths**—Stop for a minute and take three deep, cleansing breaths. Close your eyes and fill up your lungs to their maximum capacity and then slowly exhale all the pent-up energy you have inside of you. These breaths will expel the negative emotions that were coming to the surface and allow you to become present in your body. Being present allows you to make better decisions.

5. **Ask What You are Truly Hungry For**—When the urge to emotionally eat arises, it is the result of some emotional response that you are not prepared or equipped to deal with in the moment, and you are simply seeking to distract yourself. Those emotions are a result of you not getting something for yourself, so the question you must ask yourself is, "What am I *really* hungry for?" It may be someone to talk to, it may be to scream

into a pillow about how your friend did you wrong or it could be a hug from your partner. Whatever it is, discover it and if it is possible to attain, then do. If it's not possible, ask yourself what you can do in the immediate moment that will buy you some time until the feelings pass. Would going for a walk help? Or what about taking a long, luxurious bath? Refer to your self-care list and have a few personal-care activities ready to go so when these instances arise, you are ready to take care of yourself immediately until the need to eat passes.

Regardless of what happens in the moments before or after emotional eating, it is essential for you to remember to be kind and cut yourself some slack. These behaviors did not come out of nowhere, and they are not going to disappear overnight. It is going to take time, patience, grace and empathy for you to fully embrace the journey to freedom from food.

Food is not the enemy, and neither are your emotions. You must learn to be okay with sitting with and facing your emotions and your responses to certain situations. As kind as you are towards others, you need to learn to be twice as nice to yourself for all you have been through. You are taking huge strides in becoming both physically and mentally healthy, and I am confident you will learn to put your feelings, emotions and needs first and give yourself the gift of happiness that comes from loving yourself and who you are at your deepest level. This kind of love is not dependent upon any outside forces but comes from a genuine respect and love for yourself that is born out of the bravery and courage it takes to face your demons head-on.

Stop and Jot #13

Label your journal entry, "All About Me." You are going to create an instructional manual where you will have all of the most important strategies, tips and reminders from this book to help you as you address and learn to manage your emotional eating. What resonates with one person might not resonate with someone else, so I want you to look back over your journal entries and answer to each of the following prompts/questions in as much detail as possible:

Stop and Jot #13 *(Continued)*

Answer in a complete sentence. Include the question in your answer. Example: "My most common emotional eating trigger is..." and then your answer.

If you feel the question does not apply to you, skip it.

- *I can remember eating emotionally as early as...*

- *These are the incidents in my childhood that contributed to me being an emotional eater...*

- *Please write this statement in your journal as a fact:*

  I acknowledge what occurred in my childhood that caused me to turn to food for support, but as an adult, I choose not to continue to use food in that way. I rewrite my eating history with food, and it serves me positively.

Stop and Jot #13 *(Continued)*

- *What are my triggers for emotional eating?*

- *How can I avoid these triggers, or make them less powerful?*

- *What are my "in the moment" strategies for when I feel tempted to eat when not hungry?*

- *What does my Take 5 strategy look like, and does it work in stopping me from eating when I'm not physically hungry?*

- *What are the self-care activities I will use to prevent episodes of emotional eating?*

- *What positive affirmations do I recite or write every day to keep myself thinking positively?*

- *How does my daily gratitude journaling help me?*

   What is the most important thing I have learned from reading this book?

The strength you have demonstrated throughout the reading of this book and your subsequent processing of the emotions surrounding emotional eating will carry you through many challenging situations. How you do one thing is how you do all things, so this courage and fortitude to uncover some personal demons is something you will carry with you and be able to apply to all areas of your life. Being able to confront your food issues will allow you to face many things in your life that have been too scary to address, and this will empower you to take control of your present and future and make it all you want it to be.

Chapter 6
Food Freedom

Whew!

That was pretty exhausting work right there, but you powered through and you can now see the light at the end of the tunnel. Freedom from food is right around the corner.

You have done a ton of work since picking up this book, and it is my hope that you feel, at the very least, that you have a better understanding of emotional eating and how it plays out in your life. Every person's situation is different, but there is always a thread of commonality that runs through the stories of those who use food to soothe instead of to just nourish.

You have the power to be free from the control food has had over you.

Life is about taking responsibility for the decisions you make, and if a situation or a circumstance isn't working for you, it is your job to make a change so that things come more into alignment for you. It is never about blaming others for what they have done to you; in every moment of every day, you have the opportunity to see situations in either a positive or negative light. Choosing to be a victim will only bring more of those kinds of instances into your life. It is time to realize the power you have in your own life and channel that energy for good and positive things instead of towards the negative.

The same goes for your relationship with food... if it hasn't been the healthiest journey up to this point, that is in the past. It is, however something you can change in this very moment by changing how you view it.

In every circumstance in your life, the best thing you can do is ask the question, "What can I learn from this situation?" Whether things turned out positive or negative, there is always something to be gleaned from every scenario. If you choose to only focus on the positive circumstances and don't choose to learn from the negative situations, you are missing out on some incredible opportunities for amazing growth and learning.

If you go through this book, have your journal, complete all of the stop and jots, process all of the things from your past and set up a plan for when emotional eating hits, and *still* you find yourself elbow-deep in a carton of Ben and Jerry's, you have not failed, nor has this book and the process described in it let you down. You just need to take those situations and ask the question, "What can I learn from this situation to help me the next time I am in this place?" If you pass on this opportunity for learning and growth, you are missing out on the human experience of evolving into the person you want to be.

Don't get hung up on "getting it" right away. This learned behavior didn't develop overnight, and it sure as heck isn't going to go away simply by reading a book. It will take time, patience, compassion, self-love, caring, kindness and a commitment to the daily work that needs to happen to improve your overall outlook on life. If you are a person who comes from a background of negativity, it is going to take time to change the thought patterns you have ingrained in your brain over the past few decades. But it is the "changing of the tapes" you play in your mind that is the game-changer that makes everything fall into place. That, in combination with self-care, will have the greatest impact on not only your relationship with food but all the relationships in your life. The most important relationship being the one you have with yourself.

Emotions are not to be avoided or ignored. Instead, you must learn to be comfortable with simply sitting with your feelings and not giving them the overwhelming power many people turn over to them. Emotions are meant to be your friend, in the same way that food is your friend and not something that needs to be feared. As you become more at ease with your connection with food, your ability to handle your emotions will improve, and you will feel a sense of empowerment and strength you have never known before.

I am eternally grateful that you had the courage to pick up this book and dive head-first into a subject that is not a comfortable one to deal with. Please know that everything you need in order to have the most amazing life is already within you, and all that needs to be done is the internal work that will allow it to flourish and shine.

Getting to a place where you love yourself and your body exactly as it is now (not what it will be like in three weeks) is the key to life content-ment. Remembering to put yourself and your needs first so you don't have to use food to serve as a replacement for the care that you really need is your first and foremost goal.

You can do it because you are strong, confident and intelligent, and you now have the skills and the process to get you to that place. Please take the time to do this for yourself. I want only the best for you as you work to have freedom with food that allows you to live your best life, feeling amazing in your own body, mind and spirit.

Conclusion

Regardless of where you are in your emotional eating journey, knowing that you are not suffering alone can be a source of solace and comfort. Know that you no longer need to suffer in silence and you now have a resource to assist you when you feel most equipped to address your issue.

I would strongly recommend reading this book a second or even a third time in order to get as much out of it as you can. With each reading, different aspects of emotional eating will resonate with you and you will be able to better absorb and process the information.

If after reading and completing all of the writing activities, and taking yourself through the step by step process outlined, you feel like you need further assistance and support with your relationship with food, I am here to help. Please reach out and let's connect and discuss your unique situation and let me guide you through the process so you can develop a new relationship with food that makes you feel good.

———————

Ways to connect

E-mail me at:
kristin@kristinjonescoaching.com

Book a FREE 30-minute Transformation Call:
https://calendly.com/kristin-jones-coaching/initial

———————

You are worth it. You can have a relationship with food that allows you to live a complete and full life. Know this is possible for you.

You are enough.

You are loved.

References

Castle, J. (2017, July 5). Why Do Kids Eat When
They're Not Hungry? Retrieved from https://
health.usnews.com/wellness/for-
parents/articles/2017-07-05/why-do-kids-
eat-when-theyre-not-hungry

Clark, P. (2018, January 25). The Power of
Forgiveness. Retrieved from https://thrive
global.com/stories/the-power-of-forgiveness-
3/

Fish, J. (2014, February 25). Tolerance, Acceptance,
Understanding. Retrieved from https://www.
psychologytoday.com/us/blog/looking-in-
the-cultural-mirror/201402/tolerance-
acceptance-understanding

Horvath, T., Misra, K., Epner, A., & Cooper, G. M.
(n.d.). Definition Of Addiction. Retrieved
from https://www.mentalhelp.net/articles/
definition-of-addiction/

James, M. (2013). 4 Steps to Release "Limiting
Beliefs" Learned From Childhood. Retrieved

from https://www.psychologytoday.com/us/
blog/focus-forgiveness/201311/4-steps-
release-limiting-beliefs-learned-childhood

Jerabek, I. (2018, April 17). How to Stop Being an
Emotional Eater. Retrieved from http://
consciouslivingtv.com/health/whats-eating-
you.html

Melemis, S. (2018). What is Addiction? Definition,
Signs, Test, Causes, Consequences. Retrieved
from https://www.addictionsandrecovery.
org/what-is-addiction.htm

Ross, A., Brooks, A., & Wallen, G. (2016, August 10).
A Different Weight Loss Experience: A
Qualitative Study Exploring the Behavioral,
Physical, and Psychosocial Changes
Associated with Yoga That Promote Weight
Loss. Retrieved from https://www.hindawi.
com/journals/ecam/2016/2914745/

Scalise, J. (2018, December 02). How Negative Self-
Talk Sabotages Your Health & Happiness.
Retrieved from https://brainspeak.com/how-
negative-self-talk-sabotages-your-health-
happiness/

Scriven, A. (2017, December 20). How to Prevent
Emotional Eating Using Yoga. Retrieved from
https://www.doyouyoga.com/how-to-
prevent-emotional-eating-using-yoga-57087/

Smith, M., Segal, J., & Segal, R. (2018). Emotional Eating. Retrieved from https://www.help guide.org/articles/diets/emotional-eating.htm/

Talmay, O. (2014, August 11). Conquer Emotional Eating With These 12 Weird Tricks. Retrieved from https://www.huffingtonpost.com/orion-talmay/conquer-emotional-eating-with-these-12-weird-tricks_b_5471268.html

Thorp, T. (2017, February 13). How to Rewrite Your Life Story. Retrieved from https://chopra.com/articles/how-to-rewrite-your-life-story

About the Author

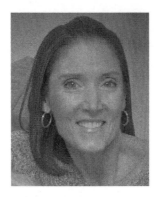

Kristin Jones is a former middle school English and History teacher-turned online wellness coach-turned best-selling author. She is the owner of Kristin Jones Coaching, an online wellness and lifestyle coaching business, where she specializes in helping women address and manage their emotional eating issues and rewrite their relationship with food. In the process, she helps each of her clients find their own unique path to lasting weight-loss success and happiness with the life they have created.

Can You Help?

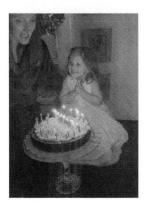

Thank You for Reading My Book!

I really appreciate all your feedback, and I love hearing what you have to say.

I need your input to make the next version of this book and my future books better.

Please leave me an honest review on Amazon letting me know what you thought of the book.

Thanks so much!
Kristin Jones

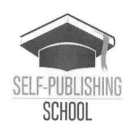

SELF-PUBLISHING
SCHOOL

NOW IT'S YOUR TURN

Discover the EXACT 3-step blueprint you need to become a bestselling author in 3 months.

Self-Publishing School helped me, and now I want them to help you with this FREE WEBINAR!

Even if you're busy, bad at writing, or don't know where to start, you CAN write a bestseller and build your best life.

With tools and experience across a variety niches and professions, Self-Publishing School is the <u>only</u> resource you need to take your book to the finish line!

DON'T WAIT

Watch this FREE WEBINAR now, and
Say "YES" to becoming a bestseller:

**https://xe172.isrefer.com/go/affegwebinar/
bookbrosinc7859/**

Made in the USA
Columbia, SC
04 February 2021